Medical Notebook

Track Your Weight, Medications,
Blood Pressure, and Blood Sugar

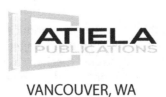

VANCOUVER, WA

Published by Atiela Publications in 2018

Design and writing © 2018 Atiela Journals

Front cover images from:
Pill Bottle: KlaraD/Shutterstock.com
Blood Pressure: natashanas/Shutterstock.com
Blood Suger: HelgaMariah/Shutterstock.com
Weight Scale: lukpedclub/Shutterstock.com

ISBN 13: 978-1-947965-02-7

My Personal Info

Name: _____

Address: _____

_____

Home Phone: _____

Cell Phone: _____

Email:_____

Date of Birth:_____

Emergency Contacts

Name: _____

Home Phone: _____

Cell Phone: _____

Relationship: _____

Name: _____

Home Phone: _____

Cell Phone: _____

Relationship: _____

Medical Contacts

Doctor: _____

Phone: _____

Dentist: _____

Phone: _____

Eye Doctor: _____

Phone: _____

Pharmacy: _____

Phone: _____

Notes

Health History

Allergies

1: _____

2: _____

3: _____

4: _____

Major Illnesses

1: _____

2: _____

3: _____

4: _____

5: _____

6: _____

Surgeries

Surgery:_____

Date of Surgery: _____

Surgery:_____

Date of Surgery: _____

Surgery:_____

Date of Surgery: _____

Surgery:_____

Date of Surgery: _____

Notes

Medicine List

Medication Name	Dose	How Often	What It's For

Notes

Medicine List

Medication Name	Dose	How Often	What It's For

Notes

Medicine List

Medication Name	Dose	How Often	What It's For

Notes

Vitamin List

Medication Name	Dose	How Often	What It's For

Weekly Log

	Mon	Tues	Wed	Thurs	Fri	Sat	Sun
Date							
Weight							
Medicines (Check off as you take them) **M = Morning | N = Noon | E = Evening | B = Bedtime**							
Took Meds	☐ M ☐ N ☐ E ☐ B	☐ M ☐ N ☐ E ☐ B	☐ M ☐ N ☐ E ☐ B	☐ M ☐ N ☐ E ☐ B	☐ M ☐ N ☐ E ☐ B	☐ M ☐ N ☐ E ☐ B	☐ M ☐ N ☐ E ☐ B
Blood Pressure							
AM							
PM							
Blood Sugar							
Break							
Snack							
Lunch							
Dinner							
Eve							

Notes

Weekly Log

	Mon	Tues	Wed	Thurs	Fri	Sat	Sun
Date							
Weight							
Medicines (Check off as you take them) M = Morning | N = Noon | E = Evening | B = Bedtime							
Took Meds	☐ M ☐ N ☐ E ☐ B	☐ M ☐ N ☐ E ☐ B	☐ M ☐ N ☐ E ☐ B	☐ M ☐ N ☐ E ☐ B	☐ M ☐ N ☐ E ☐ B	☐ M ☐ N ☐ E ☐ B	☐ M ☐ N ☐ E ☐ B
Blood Pressure							
AM							
PM							
Blood Sugar							
Break							
Snack							
Lunch							
Dinner							
Eve							

Notes

Weekly Log

	Mon	Tues	Wed	Thurs	Fri	Sat	Sun
Date							
Weight							
Medicines (Check off as you take them) M = Morning | N = Noon | E = Evening | B = Bedtime							
Took Meds	☐ M ☐ N ☐ E ☐ B	☐ M ☐ N ☐ E ☐ B	☐ M ☐ N ☐ E ☐ B	☐ M ☐ N ☐ E ☐ B	☐ M ☐ N ☐ E ☐ B	☐ M ☐ N ☐ E ☐ B	☐ M ☐ N ☐ E ☐ B
Blood Pressure							
AM							
PM							
Blood Sugar							
Break							
Snack							
Lunch							
Dinner							
Eve							

Notes

Weekly Log

	Mon	Tues	Wed	Thurs	Fri	Sat	Sun
Date							
Weight							
Medicines (Check off as you take them) M = Morning | N = Noon | E = Evening | B = Bedtime							
Took Meds	☐ M ☐ N ☐ E ☐ B	☐ M ☐ N ☐ E ☐ B	☐ M ☐ N ☐ E ☐ B	☐ M ☐ N ☐ E ☐ B	☐ M ☐ N ☐ E ☐ B	☐ M ☐ N ☐ E ☐ B	☐ M ☐ N ☐ E ☐ B
Blood Pressure							
AM							
PM							
Blood Sugar							
Break							
Snack							
Lunch							
Dinner							
Eve							

Notes

Weekly Log

	Mon	Tues	Wed	Thurs	Fri	Sat	Sun
Date							
Weight							
Medicines (Check off as you take them) M = Morning | N = Noon | E = Evening | B = Bedtime							
Took Meds	☐ M ☐ N ☐ E ☐ B	☐ M ☐ N ☐ E ☐ B	☐ M ☐ N ☐ E ☐ B	☐ M ☐ N ☐ E ☐ B	☐ M ☐ N ☐ E ☐ B	☐ M ☐ N ☐ E ☐ B	☐ M ☐ N ☐ E ☐ B
Blood Pressure							
AM							
PM							
Blood Sugar							
Break							
Snack							
Lunch							
Dinner							
Eve							

Notes

Weekly Log

	Mon	Tues	Wed	Thurs	Fri	Sat	Sun
Date							
Weight							
Medicines (Check off as you take them) M = Morning | N = Noon | E = Evening | B = Bedtime							
Took Meds	☐ M ☐ N ☐ E ☐ B	☐ M ☐ N ☐ E ☐ B	☐ M ☐ N ☐ E ☐ B	☐ M ☐ N ☐ E ☐ B	☐ M ☐ N ☐ E ☐ B	☐ M ☐ N ☐ E ☐ B	☐ M ☐ N ☐ E ☐ B
Blood Pressure							
AM							
PM							
Blood Sugar							
Break							
Snack							
Lunch							
Dinner							
Eve							

Notes

Weekly Log

	Mon	Tues	Wed	Thurs	Fri	Sat	Sun
Date							
Weight							
Medicines (Check off as you take them) M = Morning | N = Noon | E = Evening | B = Bedtime							
Took Meds	☐ M ☐ N ☐ E ☐ B	☐ M ☐ N ☐ E ☐ B	☐ M ☐ N ☐ E ☐ B	☐ M ☐ N ☐ E ☐ B	☐ M ☐ N ☐ E ☐ B	☐ M ☐ N ☐ E ☐ B	☐ M ☐ N ☐ E ☐ B
Blood Pressure							
AM							
PM							
Blood Sugar							
Break							
Snack							
Lunch							
Dinner							
Eve							

Notes

Weekly Log

	Mon	Tues	Wed	Thurs	Fri	Sat	Sun
Date							
Weight							
Medicines (Check off as you take them) M = Morning | N = Noon | E = Evening | B = Bedtime							
Took Meds	☐ M ☐ N ☐ E ☐ B	☐ M ☐ N ☐ E ☐ B	☐ M ☐ N ☐ E ☐ B	☐ M ☐ N ☐ E ☐ B	☐ M ☐ N ☐ E ☐ B	☐ M ☐ N ☐ E ☐ B	☐ M ☐ N ☐ E ☐ B
Blood Pressure							
AM							
PM							
Blood Sugar							
Break							
Snack							
Lunch							
Dinner							
Eve							

Notes

Weekly Log

	Mon	Tues	Wed	Thurs	Fri	Sat	Sun
Date							
Weight							
Medicines (Check off as you take them) M = Morning | N = Noon | E = Evening | B = Bedtime							
Took Meds	☐ M ☐ N ☐ E ☐ B	☐ M ☐ N ☐ E ☐ B	☐ M ☐ N ☐ E ☐ B	☐ M ☐ N ☐ E ☐ B	☐ M ☐ N ☐ E ☐ B	☐ M ☐ N ☐ E ☐ B	☐ M ☐ N ☐ E ☐ B
Blood Pressure							
AM							
PM							
Blood Sugar							
Break							
Snack							
Lunch							
Dinner							
Eve							

Notes

Weekly Log

	Mon	Tues	Wed	Thurs	Fri	Sat	Sun
Date							
Weight							
Medicines (Check off as you take them) M = Morning | N = Noon | E = Evening | B = Bedtime							
Took Meds	☐ M ☐ N ☐ E ☐ B	☐ M ☐ N ☐ E ☐ B	☐ M ☐ N ☐ E ☐ B	☐ M ☐ N ☐ E ☐ B	☐ M ☐ N ☐ E ☐ B	☐ M ☐ N ☐ E ☐ B	☐ M ☐ N ☐ E ☐ B
Blood Pressure							
AM							
PM							
Blood Sugar							
Break							
Snack							
Lunch							
Dinner							
Eve							

Notes

Weekly Log

	Mon	Tues	Wed	Thurs	Fri	Sat	Sun
Date							
Weight							
Medicines (Check off as you take them) M = Morning | N = Noon | E = Evening | B = Bedtime							
Took Meds	☐ M ☐ N ☐ E ☐ B	☐ M ☐ N ☐ E ☐ B	☐ M ☐ N ☐ E ☐ B	☐ M ☐ N ☐ E ☐ B	☐ M ☐ N ☐ E ☐ B	☐ M ☐ N ☐ E ☐ B	☐ M ☐ N ☐ E ☐ B
Blood Pressure							
AM							
PM							
Blood Sugar							
Break							
Snack							
Lunch							
Dinner							
Eve							

Notes

Weekly Log

	Mon	Tues	Wed	Thurs	Fri	Sat	Sun
Date							
Weight							
Medicines (Check off as you take them) M = Morning | N = Noon | E = Evening | B = Bedtime							
Took Meds	☐ M ☐ N ☐ E ☐ B	☐ M ☐ N ☐ E ☐ B	☐ M ☐ N ☐ E ☐ B	☐ M ☐ N ☐ E ☐ B	☐ M ☐ N ☐ E ☐ B	☐ M ☐ N ☐ E ☐ B	☐ M ☐ N ☐ E ☐ B
Blood Pressure							
AM							
PM							
Blood Sugar							
Break							
Snack							
Lunch							
Dinner							
Eve							

Notes

Weekly Log

	Mon	Tues	Wed	Thurs	Fri	Sat	Sun
Date							
Weight							
Medicines (Check off as you take them) M = Morning | N = Noon | E = Evening | B = Bedtime							
Took Meds	☐ M ☐ N ☐ E ☐ B	☐ M ☐ N ☐ E ☐ B	☐ M ☐ N ☐ E ☐ B	☐ M ☐ N ☐ E ☐ B	☐ M ☐ N ☐ E ☐ B	☐ M ☐ N ☐ E ☐ B	☐ M ☐ N ☐ E ☐ B
Blood Pressure							
AM							
PM							
Blood Sugar							
Break							
Snack							
Lunch							
Dinner							
Eve							

Notes

Weekly Log

	Mon	Tues	Wed	Thurs	Fri	Sat	Sun
Date							
Weight							
Medicines (Check off as you take them) M = Morning | N = Noon | E = Evening | B = Bedtime							
Took Meds	☐ M ☐ N ☐ E ☐ B	☐ M ☐ N ☐ E ☐ B	☐ M ☐ N ☐ E ☐ B	☐ M ☐ N ☐ E ☐ B	☐ M ☐ N ☐ E ☐ B	☐ M ☐ N ☐ E ☐ B	☐ M ☐ N ☐ E ☐ B
Blood Pressure							
AM							
PM							
Blood Sugar							
Break							
Snack							
Lunch							
Dinner							
Eve							

Notes

Weekly Log

	Mon	Tues	Wed	Thurs	Fri	Sat	Sun
Date							
Weight							
Medicines (Check off as you take them) M = Morning | N = Noon | E = Evening | B = Bedtime							
Took Meds	☐ M ☐ N ☐ E ☐ B	☐ M ☐ N ☐ E ☐ B	☐ M ☐ N ☐ E ☐ B	☐ M ☐ N ☐ E ☐ B	☐ M ☐ N ☐ E ☐ B	☐ M ☐ N ☐ E ☐ B	☐ M ☐ N ☐ E ☐ B
Blood Pressure							
AM							
PM							
Blood Sugar							
Break							
Snack							
Lunch							
Dinner							
Eve							

Notes

Weekly Log

	Mon	Tues	Wed	Thurs	Fri	Sat	Sun
Date							
Weight							
Medicines (Check off as you take them) M = Morning | N = Noon | E = Evening | B = Bedtime							
Took Meds	☐ M ☐ N ☐ E ☐ B	☐ M ☐ N ☐ E ☐ B	☐ M ☐ N ☐ E ☐ B	☐ M ☐ N ☐ E ☐ B	☐ M ☐ N ☐ E ☐ B	☐ M ☐ N ☐ E ☐ B	☐ M ☐ N ☐ E ☐ B
Blood Pressure							
AM							
PM							
Blood Sugar							
Break							
Snack							
Lunch							
Dinner							
Eve							

Notes

Weekly Log

	Mon	Tues	Wed	Thurs	Fri	Sat	Sun
Date							
Weight							
Medicines (Check off as you take them) M = Morning | N = Noon | E = Evening | B = Bedtime							
Took Meds	☐ M ☐ N ☐ E ☐ B	☐ M ☐ N ☐ E ☐ B	☐ M ☐ N ☐ E ☐ B	☐ M ☐ N ☐ E ☐ B	☐ M ☐ N ☐ E ☐ B	☐ M ☐ N ☐ E ☐ B	☐ M ☐ N ☐ E ☐ B
Blood Pressure							
AM							
PM							
Blood Sugar							
Break							
Snack							
Lunch							
Dinner							
Eve							

Notes

Weekly Log

	Mon	Tues	Wed	Thurs	Fri	Sat	Sun
Date							
Weight							
Medicines (Check off as you take them) M = Morning | N = Noon | E = Evening | B = Bedtime							
Took Meds	☐ M ☐ N ☐ E ☐ B	☐ M ☐ N ☐ E ☐ B	☐ M ☐ N ☐ E ☐ B	☐ M ☐ N ☐ E ☐ B	☐ M ☐ N ☐ E ☐ B	☐ M ☐ N ☐ E ☐ B	☐ M ☐ N ☐ E ☐ B
Blood Pressure							
AM							
PM							
Blood Sugar							
Break							
Snack							
Lunch							
Dinner							
Eve							

Notes

Weekly Log

	Mon	Tues	Wed	Thurs	Fri	Sat	Sun
Date							
Weight							
Medicines (Check off as you take them) M = Morning | N = Noon | E = Evening | B = Bedtime							
Took Meds	☐ M ☐ N ☐ E ☐ B	☐ M ☐ N ☐ E ☐ B	☐ M ☐ N ☐ E ☐ B	☐ M ☐ N ☐ E ☐ B	☐ M ☐ N ☐ E ☐ B	☐ M ☐ N ☐ E ☐ B	☐ M ☐ N ☐ E ☐ B
Blood Pressure							
AM							
PM							
Blood Sugar							
Break							
Snack							
Lunch							
Dinner							
Eve							

Notes

Weekly Log

	Mon	Tues	Wed	Thurs	Fri	Sat	Sun
Date							
Weight							
Medicines (Check off as you take them) M = Morning | N = Noon | E = Evening | B = Bedtime							
Took Meds	☐ M ☐ N ☐ E ☐ B	☐ M ☐ N ☐ E ☐ B	☐ M ☐ N ☐ E ☐ B	☐ M ☐ N ☐ E ☐ B	☐ M ☐ N ☐ E ☐ B	☐ M ☐ N ☐ E ☐ B	☐ M ☐ N ☐ E ☐ B
Blood Pressure							
AM							
PM							
Blood Sugar							
Break							
Snack							
Lunch							
Dinner							
Eve							

Notes

Weekly Log

	Mon	Tues	Wed	Thurs	Fri	Sat	Sun
Date							
Weight							
Medicines (Check off as you take them) M = Morning | N = Noon | E = Evening | B = Bedtime							
Took Meds	☐ M ☐ N ☐ E ☐ B	☐ M ☐ N ☐ E ☐ B	☐ M ☐ N ☐ E ☐ B	☐ M ☐ N ☐ E ☐ B	☐ M ☐ N ☐ E ☐ B	☐ M ☐ N ☐ E ☐ B	☐ M ☐ N ☐ E ☐ B
Blood Pressure							
AM							
PM							
Blood Sugar							
Break							
Snack							
Lunch							
Dinner							
Eve							

Notes

Weekly Log

	Mon	Tues	Wed	Thurs	Fri	Sat	Sun
Date							
Weight							
Medicines (Check off as you take them) **M = Morning	N = Noon	E = Evening	B = Bedtime**							
Took Meds	☐ M ☐ N ☐ E ☐ B	☐ M ☐ N ☐ E ☐ B	☐ M ☐ N ☐ E ☐ B	☐ M ☐ N ☐ E ☐ B	☐ M ☐ N ☐ E ☐ B	☐ M ☐ N ☐ E ☐ B	☐ M ☐ N ☐ E ☐ B
Blood Pressure							
AM							
PM							
Blood Sugar							
Break							
Snack							
Lunch							
Dinner							
Eve							

Notes

Weekly Log

	Mon	Tues	Wed	Thurs	Fri	Sat	Sun
Date							
Weight							
Medicines (Check off as you take them) M = Morning | N = Noon | E = Evening | B = Bedtime							
Took Meds	☐ M ☐ N ☐ E ☐ B	☐ M ☐ N ☐ E ☐ B	☐ M ☐ N ☐ E ☐ B	☐ M ☐ N ☐ E ☐ B	☐ M ☐ N ☐ E ☐ B	☐ M ☐ N ☐ E ☐ B	☐ M ☐ N ☐ E ☐ B
Blood Pressure							
AM							
PM							
Blood Sugar							
Break							
Snack							
Lunch							
Dinner							
Eve							

Notes

Weekly Log

	Mon	Tues	Wed	Thurs	Fri	Sat	Sun
Date							
Weight							
Medicines (Check off as you take them) M = Morning | N = Noon | E = Evening | B = Bedtime							
Took Meds	☐ M ☐ N ☐ E ☐ B	☐ M ☐ N ☐ E ☐ B	☐ M ☐ N ☐ E ☐ B	☐ M ☐ N ☐ E ☐ B	☐ M ☐ N ☐ E ☐ B	☐ M ☐ N ☐ E ☐ B	☐ M ☐ N ☐ E ☐ B
Blood Pressure							
AM							
PM							
Blood Sugar							
Break							
Snack							
Lunch							
Dinner							
Eve							

Notes

Weekly Log

	Mon	Tues	Wed	Thurs	Fri	Sat	Sun
Date							
Weight							
Medicines (Check off as you take them) M = Morning | N = Noon | E = Evening | B = Bedtime							
Took Meds	☐ M ☐ N ☐ E ☐ B	☐ M ☐ N ☐ E ☐ B	☐ M ☐ N ☐ E ☐ B	☐ M ☐ N ☐ E ☐ B	☐ M ☐ N ☐ E ☐ B	☐ M ☐ N ☐ E ☐ B	☐ M ☐ N ☐ E ☐ B
Blood Pressure							
AM							
PM							
Blood Sugar							
Break							
Snack							
Lunch							
Dinner							
Eve							

Notes

Weekly Log

	Mon	Tues	Wed	Thurs	Fri	Sat	Sun
Date							
Weight							
Medicines (Check off as you take them) M = Morning | N = Noon | E = Evening | B = Bedtime							
Took Meds	☐ M ☐ N ☐ E ☐ B	☐ M ☐ N ☐ E ☐ B	☐ M ☐ N ☐ E ☐ B	☐ M ☐ N ☐ E ☐ B	☐ M ☐ N ☐ E ☐ B	☐ M ☐ N ☐ E ☐ B	☐ M ☐ N ☐ E ☐ B
Blood Pressure							
AM							
PM							
Blood Sugar							
Break							
Snack							
Lunch							
Dinner							
Eve							

Notes

Weekly Log

	Mon	Tues	Wed	Thurs	Fri	Sat	Sun
Date							
Weight							
Medicines (Check off as you take them) M = Morning | N = Noon | E = Evening | B = Bedtime							
Took Meds	☐ M ☐ N ☐ E ☐ B	☐ M ☐ N ☐ E ☐ B	☐ M ☐ N ☐ E ☐ B	☐ M ☐ N ☐ E ☐ B	☐ M ☐ N ☐ E ☐ B	☐ M ☐ N ☐ E ☐ B	☐ M ☐ N ☐ E ☐ B
Blood Pressure							
AM							
PM							
Blood Sugar							
Break							
Snack							
Lunch							
Dinner							
Eve							

Notes

Weekly Log

	Mon	Tues	Wed	Thurs	Fri	Sat	Sun
Date							
Weight							
Medicines (Check off as you take them) M = Morning | N = Noon | E = Evening | B = Bedtime							
Took Meds	☐ M ☐ N ☐ E ☐ B	☐ M ☐ N ☐ E ☐ B	☐ M ☐ N ☐ E ☐ B	☐ M ☐ N ☐ E ☐ B	☐ M ☐ N ☐ E ☐ B	☐ M ☐ N ☐ E ☐ B	☐ M ☐ N ☐ E ☐ B
Blood Pressure							
AM							
PM							
Blood Sugar							
Break							
Snack							
Lunch							
Dinner							
Eve							

Notes

Weekly Log

	Mon	Tues	Wed	Thurs	Fri	Sat	Sun
Date							
Weight							
Medicines (Check off as you take them) M = Morning | N = Noon | E = Evening | B = Bedtime							
Took Meds	☐ M ☐ N ☐ E ☐ B	☐ M ☐ N ☐ E ☐ B	☐ M ☐ N ☐ E ☐ B	☐ M ☐ N ☐ E ☐ B	☐ M ☐ N ☐ E ☐ B	☐ M ☐ N ☐ E ☐ B	☐ M ☐ N ☐ E ☐ B
Blood Pressure							
AM							
PM							
Blood Sugar							
Break							
Snack							
Lunch							
Dinner							
Eve							

Notes

Weekly Log

	Mon	Tues	Wed	Thurs	Fri	Sat	Sun
Date							
Weight							
Medicines (Check off as you take them) **M = Morning | N = Noon | E = Evening | B = Bedtime**							
Took Meds	☐ M ☐ N ☐ E ☐ B	☐ M ☐ N ☐ E ☐ B	☐ M ☐ N ☐ E ☐ B	☐ M ☐ N ☐ E ☐ B	☐ M ☐ N ☐ E ☐ B	☐ M ☐ N ☐ E ☐ B	☐ M ☐ N ☐ E ☐ B
Blood Pressure							
AM							
PM							
Blood Sugar							
Break							
Snack							
Lunch							
Dinner							
Eve							

Notes

Weekly Log

	Mon	Tues	Wed	Thurs	Fri	Sat	Sun
Date							
Weight							
Medicines (Check off as you take them) M = Morning | N = Noon | E = Evening | B = Bedtime							
Took Meds	☐ M ☐ N ☐ E ☐ B	☐ M ☐ N ☐ E ☐ B	☐ M ☐ N ☐ E ☐ B	☐ M ☐ N ☐ E ☐ B	☐ M ☐ N ☐ E ☐ B	☐ M ☐ N ☐ E ☐ B	☐ M ☐ N ☐ E ☐ B
Blood Pressure							
AM							
PM							
Blood Sugar							
Break							
Snack							
Lunch							
Dinner							
Eve							

Notes

Weekly Log

	Mon	Tues	Wed	Thurs	Fri	Sat	Sun
Date							
Weight							
Medicines (Check off as you take them) M = Morning | N = Noon | E = Evening | B = Bedtime							
Took Meds	☐ M ☐ N ☐ E ☐ B	☐ M ☐ N ☐ E ☐ B	☐ M ☐ N ☐ E ☐ B	☐ M ☐ N ☐ E ☐ B	☐ M ☐ N ☐ E ☐ B	☐ M ☐ N ☐ E ☐ B	☐ M ☐ N ☐ E ☐ B
Blood Pressure							
AM							
PM							
Blood Sugar							
Break							
Snack							
Lunch							
Dinner							
Eve							

Notes

Weekly Log

	Mon	Tues	Wed	Thurs	Fri	Sat	Sun
Date							
Weight							
Medicines (Check off as you take them) M = Morning | N = Noon | E = Evening | B = Bedtime							
Took Meds	☐ M ☐ N ☐ E ☐ B	☐ M ☐ N ☐ E ☐ B	☐ M ☐ N ☐ E ☐ B	☐ M ☐ N ☐ E ☐ B	☐ M ☐ N ☐ E ☐ B	☐ M ☐ N ☐ E ☐ B	☐ M ☐ N ☐ E ☐ B
Blood Pressure							
AM							
PM							
Blood Sugar							
Break							
Snack							
Lunch							
Dinner							
Eve							

Notes

Weekly Log

	Mon	Tues	Wed	Thurs	Fri	Sat	Sun
Date							
Weight							
Medicines (Check off as you take them) M = Morning | N = Noon | E = Evening | B = Bedtime							
Took Meds	☐ M ☐ N ☐ E ☐ B	☐ M ☐ N ☐ E ☐ B	☐ M ☐ N ☐ E ☐ B	☐ M ☐ N ☐ E ☐ B	☐ M ☐ N ☐ E ☐ B	☐ M ☐ N ☐ E ☐ B	☐ M ☐ N ☐ E ☐ B
Blood Pressure							
AM							
PM							
Blood Sugar							
Break							
Snack							
Lunch							
Dinner							
Eve							

Notes

Weekly Log

	Mon	Tues	Wed	Thurs	Fri	Sat	Sun
Date							
Weight							
Medicines (Check off as you take them) M = Morning | N = Noon | E = Evening | B = Bedtime							
Took Meds	☐ M ☐ N ☐ E ☐ B	☐ M ☐ N ☐ E ☐ B	☐ M ☐ N ☐ E ☐ B	☐ M ☐ N ☐ E ☐ B	☐ M ☐ N ☐ E ☐ B	☐ M ☐ N ☐ E ☐ B	☐ M ☐ N ☐ E ☐ B
Blood Pressure							
AM							
PM							
Blood Sugar							
Break							
Snack							
Lunch							
Dinner							
Eve							

Notes

Weekly Log

	Mon	Tues	Wed	Thurs	Fri	Sat	Sun
Date							
Weight							
Medicines (Check off as you take them) **M = Morning | N = Noon | E = Evening | B = Bedtime**							
Took Meds	☐ M ☐ N ☐ E ☐ B	☐ M ☐ N ☐ E ☐ B	☐ M ☐ N ☐ E ☐ B	☐ M ☐ N ☐ E ☐ B	☐ M ☐ N ☐ E ☐ B	☐ M ☐ N ☐ E ☐ B	☐ M ☐ N ☐ E ☐ B
Blood Pressure							
AM							
PM							
Blood Sugar							
Break							
Snack							
Lunch							
Dinner							
Eve							

Notes

Weekly Log

	Mon	Tues	Wed	Thurs	Fri	Sat	Sun
Date							
Weight							
Medicines (Check off as you take them) M = Morning | N = Noon | E = Evening | B = Bedtime							
Took Meds	☐ M ☐ N ☐ E ☐ B	☐ M ☐ N ☐ E ☐ B	☐ M ☐ N ☐ E ☐ B	☐ M ☐ N ☐ E ☐ B	☐ M ☐ N ☐ E ☐ B	☐ M ☐ N ☐ E ☐ B	☐ M ☐ N ☐ E ☐ B
Blood Pressure							
AM							
PM							
Blood Sugar							
Break							
Snack							
Lunch							
Dinner							
Eve							

Notes

Weekly Log

	Mon	Tues	Wed	Thurs	Fri	Sat	Sun
Date							
Weight							
Medicines (Check off as you take them) M = Morning | N = Noon | E = Evening | B = Bedtime							
Took Meds	☐ M ☐ N ☐ E ☐ B	☐ M ☐ N ☐ E ☐ B	☐ M ☐ N ☐ E ☐ B	☐ M ☐ N ☐ E ☐ B	☐ M ☐ N ☐ E ☐ B	☐ M ☐ N ☐ E ☐ B	☐ M ☐ N ☐ E ☐ B
Blood Pressure							
AM							
PM							
Blood Sugar							
Break							
Snack							
Lunch							
Dinner							
Eve							

Notes

Weekly Log

	Mon	Tues	Wed	Thurs	Fri	Sat	Sun
Date							
Weight							
Medicines (Check off as you take them) M = Morning | N = Noon | E = Evening | B = Bedtime							
Took Meds	☐ M ☐ N ☐ E ☐ B	☐ M ☐ N ☐ E ☐ B	☐ M ☐ N ☐ E ☐ B	☐ M ☐ N ☐ E ☐ B	☐ M ☐ N ☐ E ☐ B	☐ M ☐ N ☐ E ☐ B	☐ M ☐ N ☐ E ☐ B
Blood Pressure							
AM							
PM							
Blood Sugar							
Break							
Snack							
Lunch							
Dinner							
Eve							

Notes

Weekly Log

	Mon	Tues	Wed	Thurs	Fri	Sat	Sun
Date							
Weight							
Medicines (Check off as you take them) M = Morning | N = Noon | E = Evening | B = Bedtime							
Took Meds	☐ M ☐ N ☐ E ☐ B	☐ M ☐ N ☐ E ☐ B	☐ M ☐ N ☐ E ☐ B	☐ M ☐ N ☐ E ☐ B	☐ M ☐ N ☐ E ☐ B	☐ M ☐ N ☐ E ☐ B	☐ M ☐ N ☐ E ☐ B
Blood Pressure							
AM							
PM							
Blood Sugar							
Break							
Snack							
Lunch							
Dinner							
Eve							

Notes

Weekly Log

	Mon	Tues	Wed	Thurs	Fri	Sat	Sun
Date							
Weight							
Medicines (Check off as you take them) M = Morning | N = Noon | E = Evening | B = Bedtime							
Took Meds	☐ M ☐ N ☐ E ☐ B	☐ M ☐ N ☐ E ☐ B	☐ M ☐ N ☐ E ☐ B	☐ M ☐ N ☐ E ☐ B	☐ M ☐ N ☐ E ☐ B	☐ M ☐ N ☐ E ☐ B	☐ M ☐ N ☐ E ☐ B
Blood Pressure							
AM							
PM							
Blood Sugar							
Break							
Snack							
Lunch							
Dinner							
Eve							

Notes

Weekly Log

	Mon	Tues	Wed	Thurs	Fri	Sat	Sun
Date							
Weight							
Medicines (Check off as you take them) **M = Morning | N = Noon | E = Evening | B = Bedtime**							
Took Meds	☐ M ☐ N ☐ E ☐ B	☐ M ☐ N ☐ E ☐ B	☐ M ☐ N ☐ E ☐ B	☐ M ☐ N ☐ E ☐ B	☐ M ☐ N ☐ E ☐ B	☐ M ☐ N ☐ E ☐ B	☐ M ☐ N ☐ E ☐ B
Blood Pressure							
AM							
PM							
Blood Sugar							
Break							
Snack							
Lunch							
Dinner							
Eve							

Notes

Weekly Log

	Mon	Tues	Wed	Thurs	Fri	Sat	Sun
Date							
Weight							
Medicines (Check off as you take them) M = Morning | N = Noon | E = Evening | B = Bedtime							
Took Meds	☐ M ☐ N ☐ E ☐ B	☐ M ☐ N ☐ E ☐ B	☐ M ☐ N ☐ E ☐ B	☐ M ☐ N ☐ E ☐ B	☐ M ☐ N ☐ E ☐ B	☐ M ☐ N ☐ E ☐ B	☐ M ☐ N ☐ E ☐ B
Blood Pressure							
AM							
PM							
Blood Sugar							
Break							
Snack							
Lunch							
Dinner							
Eve							

Notes

Weekly Log

	Mon	Tues	Wed	Thurs	Fri	Sat	Sun
Date							
Weight							
Medicines (Check off as you take them) M = Morning | N = Noon | E = Evening | B = Bedtime							
Took Meds	☐ M ☐ N ☐ E ☐ B	☐ M ☐ N ☐ E ☐ B	☐ M ☐ N ☐ E ☐ B	☐ M ☐ N ☐ E ☐ B	☐ M ☐ N ☐ E ☐ B	☐ M ☐ N ☐ E ☐ B	☐ M ☐ N ☐ E ☐ B
Blood Pressure							
AM							
PM							
Blood Sugar							
Break							
Snack							
Lunch							
Dinner							
Eve							

Notes

Weekly Log

	Mon	Tues	Wed	Thurs	Fri	Sat	Sun
Date							
Weight							
Medicines (Check off as you take them) M = Morning | N = Noon | E = Evening | B = Bedtime							
Took Meds	☐ M ☐ N ☐ E ☐ B	☐ M ☐ N ☐ E ☐ B	☐ M ☐ N ☐ E ☐ B	☐ M ☐ N ☐ E ☐ B	☐ M ☐ N ☐ E ☐ B	☐ M ☐ N ☐ E ☐ B	☐ M ☐ N ☐ E ☐ B
Blood Pressure							
AM							
PM							
Blood Sugar							
Break							
Snack							
Lunch							
Dinner							
Eve							

Notes

Weekly Log

	Mon	Tues	Wed	Thurs	Fri	Sat	Sun
Date							
Weight							
Medicines (Check off as you take them) M = Morning | N = Noon | E = Evening | B = Bedtime							
Took Meds	☐ M ☐ N ☐ E ☐ B	☐ M ☐ N ☐ E ☐ B	☐ M ☐ N ☐ E ☐ B	☐ M ☐ N ☐ E ☐ B	☐ M ☐ N ☐ E ☐ B	☐ M ☐ N ☐ E ☐ B	☐ M ☐ N ☐ E ☐ B
Blood Pressure							
AM							
PM							
Blood Sugar							
Break							
Snack							
Lunch							
Dinner							
Eve							

Notes

Weekly Log

	Mon	Tues	Wed	Thurs	Fri	Sat	Sun
Date							
Weight							
Medicines (Check off as you take them) M = Morning | N = Noon | E = Evening | B = Bedtime							
Took Meds	☐ M ☐ N ☐ E ☐ B	☐ M ☐ N ☐ E ☐ B	☐ M ☐ N ☐ E ☐ B	☐ M ☐ N ☐ E ☐ B	☐ M ☐ N ☐ E ☐ B	☐ M ☐ N ☐ E ☐ B	☐ M ☐ N ☐ E ☐ B
Blood Pressure							
AM							
PM							
Blood Sugar							
Break							
Snack							
Lunch							
Dinner							
Eve							

Notes

Weekly Log

	Mon	Tues	Wed	Thurs	Fri	Sat	Sun
Date							
Weight							
Medicines (Check off as you take them) M = Morning | N = Noon | E = Evening | B = Bedtime							
Took Meds	☐ M ☐ N ☐ E ☐ B	☐ M ☐ N ☐ E ☐ B	☐ M ☐ N ☐ E ☐ B	☐ M ☐ N ☐ E ☐ B	☐ M ☐ N ☐ E ☐ B	☐ M ☐ N ☐ E ☐ B	☐ M ☐ N ☐ E ☐ B
Blood Pressure							
AM							
PM							
Blood Sugar							
Break							
Snack							
Lunch							
Dinner							
Eve							

Notes

Weekly Log

	Mon	Tues	Wed	Thurs	Fri	Sat	Sun
Date							
Weight							
Medicines (Check off as you take them) M = Morning | N = Noon | E = Evening | B = Bedtime							
Took Meds	☐ M ☐ N ☐ E ☐ B	☐ M ☐ N ☐ E ☐ B	☐ M ☐ N ☐ E ☐ B	☐ M ☐ N ☐ E ☐ B	☐ M ☐ N ☐ E ☐ B	☐ M ☐ N ☐ E ☐ B	☐ M ☐ N ☐ E ☐ B
Blood Pressure							
AM							
PM							
Blood Sugar							
Break							
Snack							
Lunch							
Dinner							
Eve							

Notes

Weekly Log

	Mon	Tues	Wed	Thurs	Fri	Sat	Sun
Date							
Weight							
Medicines (Check off as you take them) **M = Morning | N = Noon | E = Evening | B = Bedtime**							
Took Meds	☐ M ☐ N ☐ E ☐ B	☐ M ☐ N ☐ E ☐ B	☐ M ☐ N ☐ E ☐ B	☐ M ☐ N ☐ E ☐ B	☐ M ☐ N ☐ E ☐ B	☐ M ☐ N ☐ E ☐ B	☐ M ☐ N ☐ E ☐ B
Blood Pressure							
AM							
PM							
Blood Sugar							
Break							
Snack							
Lunch							
Dinner							
Eve							

Notes

Weekly Log

	Mon	Tues	Wed	Thurs	Fri	Sat	Sun
Date							
Weight							
Medicines (Check off as you take them) M = Morning | N = Noon | E = Evening | B = Bedtime							
Took Meds	☐ M ☐ N ☐ E ☐ B	☐ M ☐ N ☐ E ☐ B	☐ M ☐ N ☐ E ☐ B	☐ M ☐ N ☐ E ☐ B	☐ M ☐ N ☐ E ☐ B	☐ M ☐ N ☐ E ☐ B	☐ M ☐ N ☐ E ☐ B
Blood Pressure							
AM							
PM							
Blood Sugar							
Break							
Snack							
Lunch							
Dinner							
Eve							

Notes

Made in the USA
Monee, IL
19 October 2023

44863078R00070